Table of Contents

INTRODUCTION

When we think of a "diet" these days, we usually think of some kind of restriction that will help us reach a specific outcome, such as weight loss. The Mediterranean diet couldn't be further from that. Rather, it encourages an eating pattern that includes the food staples of people who live in the countries around the Mediterranean Sea, such as Spain, Greece, Italy and France.right up arrow It also focuses on community when eating — think meals with family and friends and enjoyable conversation.right up arrow. You'll find that in their meals, Mediterranean dieters emphasize a plant-based eating approach loaded with vegetables and healthy fats, including olive oil and omega-3 fatty acids from fish.

It's a diet known for being heart-healthy.right up arrow. Eating this way means you also have little room for processed fare. When you look at a plate, it should be bursting with color; traditional proteins like chicken may be more of a side dish compared with produce, which becomes the main event. One thing you'll find people love about the

Mediterranean diet is the allowance of low to moderate amounts of red wine. "Moderate" means 5 ounces (oz) or less each day (that's around one glass). It's worth noting, though, that a daily glass of wine is not mandatory on this eating plan, and if you don't already drink, this allowance isn't a directive to start.

WHAT FOODS CAN'T YOU EAT ON THE MEDITERRANEAN DIET?

No food is banned, but the Mediterranean diet encourages limiting foods, such as red meat and sugary foods. Consume poultry, eggs, cheese, and yogurt moderately. In addition, most of the time, avoid soda, highly processed foods, and processed meats.

What's an example of a Mediterranean diet breakfast?

Is oatmeal okay on the Mediterranean diet? What about cheese? Bananas?

If I'm on the Mediterranean diet, what can I put in my coffee?

What bread can you eat on the Mediterranean diet?

How Does the Mediterranean Diet Work?

Because it wasn't developed ad hoc but is a style of eating in a region of people that evolved naturally over centuries, there's no official way to follow the Mediterranean diet. It's popular because it's a well-rounded approach to eating that isn't restrictive. Also worth noting is that two of the five so-called blue zones — areas where people live longer and have lower rates of disease — are located in Mediterranean cities (Ikaria in Greece and Sardinia in Italy).right up arrow

Potential Health Benefits of the Mediterranean Diet

The Mediterranean diet is famous for its touted health benefits, which may be attributed to its high produce content. Indeed, people typically eat three to nine servings of vegetables and up to two servings of fruit a day on a Mediterranean diet.right up arrow These fresh, whole foods pack an array of disease-fighting antioxidants, and people who fill their diet with these foods have a lower risk of disease. Yet scientists don't know if it's the antioxidants or other compounds (or general healthy eating patterns) that are responsible for these advantages.right up arrow. Here's a snapshot of some possible Mediterranean diet health benefits.

A Healthier Heart

This eating approach may be most famous for its benefit to heart health, decreasing the risk of heart disease by, in part, lowering levels of cholesterolright up arrow and reducing mortality from cardiovascular conditions.right up arrow

A Reduced Risk for Certain Cancers

Similarly, the Mediterranean diet has been linked with a lower likelihood of certain cancers,right up arrow such as breast cancer,right up arrow colon cancer,right up arrow prostate cancer,right up arrow and some head and neck cancers.right up arrow

A Sunnier Mood and a Lower Risk of Depression

If eating in the Mediterranean style prompts you to consume more fruit and vegetables, you'll not only feel better physically, but your mental health will get a lift, too. Research shows that people who eat more raw fruit and veggies (particularly dark leafy greens like spinach, fresh berries, and cucumber) have fewer symptoms of depression, a better mood, and more life satisfaction.right up arrow Other research, published in Clinical Practice &

Epidemiology in Mental Health in July 2020, suggests a Mediterranean eating style can support mental health and may play a role in reducing symptoms of depression.

A Lower Risk of Neurodegenerative Diseases

Research has found that a Mediterranean-style diet is associated with better measures of general cognitive function.right up arrow Over time, the eating pattern may slow cognitive decline and lower the risk of Alzheimer's disease and other forms of dementia.right up arrow

A Reduced Type 2 Diabetes Risk and Better Diabetes Management

Emerging evidence suggests that eating this way offers protective effects for those who have or are at risk for type 2 diabetes. For one thing, Mediterranean eating improves blood sugar control in those who already have diabetes, suggesting it can be a good way to manage the disease, according to a review of research.right up arrow What's more, given that those with diabetes are at increased odds for cardiovascular disease, adopting this diet can help improve their heart health, according to research.right up arrow

As a traditional way of eating for many cultures worldwide, the Mediterranean diet wasn't designed for weight loss. It just so happens that one of the healthiest diets around the globe is also good for keeping your weight down.

One review looked at five trials on overweight and obese people and found that after one year those who followed a Mediterranean diet lost as much as 11 pounds (lb) more than low-fat eaters.right up arrow (They dropped between 9 and 22 lb total and kept it off for a year.) But that same study found similar weight loss in other diets, like low-carb diets and the American Diabetes Association diet. The results suggest, the researchers say, that "there is no ideal diet for achieving sustained weight loss in overweight or obese individuals."

Yet a Mediterranean diet can be a varied and inclusive way to lose weight that ditches gimmicks and doesn't require calorie or macronutrient counting they way other diets (looking at you, ketogenic diet) do. And with the emphasis on healthy fat, it's satisfying, too. That said, in 2022 U.S. News & World Report ranked the Mediterranean diet No. 1

in the category Best Diets Overall and 12 in its list of Best Weight-Loss Diets.right up arrow

It's not a slam dunk, researchers note, and instead depends on how you eat. Portion sizes and fat amounts matter even in healthy diets like the Mediterranean.

A DETAILED MEDITERRANEAN DIET FOOD LIST

On the Mediterranean diet, you'll rely heavily on the following foods and limit those that are processed. Examples of processed foods include cold cuts and sausage (and other processed meats), salty packaged snacks like potato chips and crackers, and prepared sweets like cookies, cake, and candy. You may choose to drink a little red wine and eat some dark chocolate. While you don't have to count calories on the Mediterranean diet, we've included nutrition information for the following foods for your reference.

Olive Oil

Per tablespoon serving 119 calories, 0 grams (g) protein, 13.5g fat, 2g saturated fat, 10g monounsaturated fat, 0g carbohydrate, 0g fiber, 0g sugarright up arrow

Benefits Replacing foods high in saturated fats (like butter) with plant sources high in monounsaturated fatty acids, like olive oil, may help lower the risk of heart disease by 19 percent, according to research.right up arrow

Tomatoes

Per 1 cup (chopped) serving 32 calories, 1.6g protein, 0g fat, 7g carbohydrates, 2g fiber, 5g sugarright up arrow

Benefits They pack lycopene, a powerful antioxidant that is associated with a reduced risk of some cancers, like prostate and breast. Other components in tomatoes may help reduce the risk of blood clots, thereby protecting against cardiovascular disease, according to a March 2019 review in Critical Reviews in Food Science and Nutrition.

Salmon

Per 1 small fillet 130 calories, 21g protein, 4.5g fat, 0g carbohydrates, 0g fiberright up arrow

Benefits The fatty fish is a major source of omega-3 fatty acids. For good heart health, eat at least two fish meals per week, particularly fatty fish like salmon.right up arrow

Walnuts

Per 1 oz (14 halves) serving 185 calories, 4g protein, 18.5g fat, 2g saturated fat, 3g monounsaturated fat, 13g polyunsaturated fat, 4g carbohydrate, 2g fiber, 1g sugarright up arrow

Benefits Rich in heart-healthy polyunsaturated fats, these nuts may also favorably impact your gut microbiome (and thus improve digestive health), as well as lower LDL cholesterol, according to a small study that included 18 healthy adults.right up arrow

Chickpeas

Per 1 cup serving 210 calories, 11g protein, 4g fat, 35g carbohydrate, 10g fiberright up arrow

Benefits The main ingredient in hummus, chickpeas are a good source of fiber,right up arrow which brings digestive health and weight loss benefits, as well as iron, zinc, folate, and magnesium.right up arrow

Arugula

Per 1 cup serving 5 calories, 0.5g protein, 0g fat, 1g carbohydrate, 0g fiber, 0g sugarright up arrow

Benefits Leafy greens, like arugula, are eaten in abundance under this eating approach. Mediterranean-like diets that include frequent (more than six times a week) consumption of leafy greens have been shown to reduce the risk of Alzheimer's disease, according to a study.right up arrow

Pomegranate

Per ½ cup serving (arils) 72 calories, 1.5g protein, 1g fat, 16g carbohydrates, 4g fiber, 12g sugarright up arrow

Benefits This fruit, in all its bright red glory, packs powerful polyphenols that act as an antioxidant and anti-inflammatory. It's been suggested that pomegranates have anticancer properties, too, according to research.right up arrow

Lentils

Per ½ cup serving 116 calories, 9g protein, 0g fat, 20g carbohydrate, 8g fiber, 2g sugarright up arrow

Benefits One small study suggested that swapping one-half of your serving of a high-glycemic starch (like rice) with lentils helps lower the glycemic response by 20 percent.right up arrow

Farro

Per ¼ cup (uncooked) serving 190 calories, 6g protein, 1g fat, 38g carbohydrate, 5g fiber, 0g sugarright up arrow

Benefits Whole grains like farro are a staple of this diet. This grain offers a stellar source of satiating fiber and protein. Whole grains are associated with a reduced risk of a host of diseases, like stroke, type 2 diabetes, heart disease, and colorectal cancer.right up arrow

Greek Yogurt

Per 7 oz container (low-fat plain) 146 calories, 20g protein, 4g fat, 2g saturated fat, 1g monounsaturated fat, 0g polyunsaturated fat, 8g carbs, 0g fiber, 7g sugarright up arrow

Benefits Dairy is eaten in limited amounts, but these foods serve to supply an excellent source of calcium. Opting for low- or nonfat versions decreases the amount of saturated fat you're consuming.right up arrow

A 7-Day Sample Mediterranean Diet Meal Plan

To get an idea of what eating on a Mediterranean diet looks like, check out this sample week of meals, including snack ideas.

Day 1

Breakfast Greek yogurt topped with berries and a drizzle of honey

Snack Handful of almonds

Lunch Tuna on a bed of greens with a vinaigrette made with olive oil

Snack Small bowl of olives

Dinner Small chicken breast over a warm grain salad made with sautéed zucchini, tomato, and farro

Day 2

Breakfast Whole-grain toast with a soft-boiled egg and a piece of fruit

Snack Handful of pistachios

Lunch Lentil salad with roasted red peppers, sun-dried tomatoes, capers, and an olive oil–based vinaigrette

Snack Hummus with dipping veggies

Dinner Salmon with quinoa and sautéed garlicky greens

Day 3

Breakfast Whipped ricotta topped with walnuts and fruit

Snack Roasted chickpeas

Lunch Tabouli salad with whole-grain pita and hummus

Snack Caprese skewers

Dinner Roasted chicken, gnocchi, and a large salad with vinaigrette

Day 4

Breakfast Fruit with a couple of slices of brie

Snack Cashews and dried fruit

Lunch Lentil soup with whole-grain roll

Snack Tasting plate with olives, a couple slices of cheese, cucumbers, and cherry tomatoes

Dinner Whitefish cooked in olive oil and garlic, spiralized zucchini, and a sweet potato

Day 5

Breakfast Omelet made with tomatoes, fresh herbs, and olives

Snack A couple of dates stuffed with almond butter

Lunch A salad topped with white beans, veggies, olives, and a small piece of chicken

Day 6

Breakfast Eggs scrambled with veggies and chives and topped with feta with a slice of whole-grain bread

Snack Greek yogurt

Lunch A quinoa bowl topped with sliced chicken, feta, and veggies

Snack Hummus with veggies

Dinner Grilled seafood, roasted fennel and broccoli, arugula salad, and quinoa

Day 7

Breakfast Veggie frittata

Snack Handful of berries

Lunch A plate of smoked salmon, capers, lemon, whole-grain crackers, and raw veggies

Snack Mashed avocado with lemon and salt, with cucumbers for dipping

Dinner Pasta with red sauce and mussels

4 TIPS FOR DINING OUT ON THE MEDITERRANEAN DIET

Heading to a restaurant? Eat the Mediterranean way — and feel satisfied with these tips.

1. Prioritize Vegetables

The Mediterranean diet emphasizes vegetables, so look for vegetable-forward dishes, which can often be found in the appetizer, side, and salad section of the menu. Another option is to start your meal with a salad or roasted vegetables.right up arrow Ask that they leave off any dressings and drizzle it with olive oil instead.

2. Order the Fish

If you like fish but struggle to eat it at home regularly, order it when you're out at a restaurant where a chef is preparing it for you. This can be especially impactful if you typically order red meat when out. Go for fatty fish that are packed with omega-3 fatty acids.right up arrow Salmon is widely available and easy to find, but you may see tuna and mackerel on the menu, too.

3. Limit Alcohol

If you drink alcohol, skip the margarita or beer and instead opt for an occasional glass of red wine, which can be consumed in moderation with your meal.right up arrow Other times, avoid alcohol altogether in favor of a sparkling plain water with a lemon or lime wedge.

4. Nosh on Fruit for Dessert

In many cultures, fresh fruit is traditionally consumed for dessert.right up arrow Most restaurants don't have fresh fruit on their dessert menu, but you can ask if they're able to bring out a small fruit cup for you to end your meal. Or, say no to the dessert entirely and head home to fix yourself a plate of berries or a few slices of melon.

5 Beginner Tips to Keep in Mind on the Mediterranean Diet

A registered dietitian-nutritionist, whom you can find at Eatright.org, can help you start and stick with the Mediterranean diet, but these tips may also be helpful.

1. Opt for Healthy Fat Sources, and Don't Go Overboard

By limiting large amounts of red or processed meats and relying heavily on foods that are good sources of monounsaturated fatty acids, like avocado, nuts, or olive oil, you'll keep saturated fat levels low.right up arrow These fats don't lead to high cholesterol the same way saturated fats do. Healthful sources of fat include olive oil, fish oils, and nut-based oils, Cohen explains.

Even with healthy fat, your total fat consumption could be greater than the daily recommended amount if you aren't careful. Aim to get 20 to 35 percent of your total daily caloric intake from fat, and for saturated fats to represent less than 10 percent of your total caloric intake, advises the U.S. Department of Health and Human Services.

2. Don't Skimp on Calcium

Cheese and yogurt provide calcium, but on the Mediterranean diet, you eat these only in moderation.

Cohen suggests seeking out nondairy sources of calcium, such as fortified almond milk, sardines, kale, and tofu made with calcium sulfate.right up arrow3. Carve Out Time in Your Schedule to Cook

While you don't have to spend hours in your kitchen, you will need to cook, because the diet is all about working with delicious fresh food. There may be a learning curve as you build these skills.

4. Edit Your Favorite Recipes to Make Them Mediterranean Diet Friendly

It's evident that with such a variety of whole, fresh foods on the table, it's easy to build meals with this diet. And you don't have to eliminate your favorites — they may just require some tweaks. For instance, rather than a sausage and pepperoni pizza, you'd choose one piled high with veggies. You can also fit a lot of different foods into one meal. Filling up on fresh fruit and vegetables will allow you to build volume into meals for fewer calories.

5. Don't Go Overboard on Alcohol

One hallmark of a Mediterranean diet is that sociable consumption of red wine is thought to be a big reason why the diet is so healthy. But women should still stick to one glass and men two glasses. If you have a history of breast cancer in the family, know that any alcohol consumption raises that risk.right up arrow In that case, talk to your doctor to find out what's right for you.

Is the Mediterranean Diet Best for Diabetes?

Research shows the heart-healthy Mediterranean diet is also beneficial for people with type 2 diabetes. Find out how this approach can improve your blood sugar and help you lose weight — and how to get started. The Mediterranean diet — which gets its name from the traditional eating and cooking patterns of people in countries bordering the Mediterranean Sea — has long been studied for its heart health benefits. But research suggests this approach can also offer specific advantages for people living with type 2 diabetes. Among them: improved blood sugar, weight loss, and satisfying and flavorful ingredients.

Overall, the Mediterranean diet offers more of the foods your body needs, such as vegetables, whole grains, and healthy fats, and less of what it doesn't, including red meat, refined carbohydrates, and sugary fare. In past research, scientists compared the Mediterranean diet with vegetarian, vegan, low-carbohydrate, high-protein, high-fiber, and low-glycemic index diets and found that the Mediterranean diet came out on top. Study participants following Mediterranean, low-glycemic index, low-carbohydrate, and high-protein diets all experienced better blood sugar control, as was indicated by their lower A1C scores. (A1C is a measure of average blood sugar levels over a three-month period.) But people following the Mediterranean diet saw significant additional benefits — they lost the most weight and saw improved cardiovascular health, including better cholesterol levels.

"The Mediterranean diet is rich in fruits and vegetables and uses whole grains and lean protein, such as fish, as well as olive oil and nuts as the sources of fat," says Betul

Hatipoglu, MD, an endocrinologist at the University Hospitals Cleveland Medical Center in Ohio. "These healthy choices make the diet very rich in monounsaturated fat and fiber, and both have been known to lower cholesterol and blood sugar in people with diabetes."

The Mediterranean diet has a host of benefits including weight loss, heart, and brain health. That's why the Mediterranean diet is known as a heart-healthy style of eating. "In diabetes, it's all about reducing your risk for having complications from the disease," says Sharon Movsas, RDN, CDCES, a clinical nutritionist and diabetes care specialist with Montefiore Health System in the Bronx, New York. "One of the leading complications is cardiovascular disease, including heart attacks and strokes," she says. If that wasn't enough, diabetes also often comes with high blood pressure and cholesterol, both factors that increases the risk of heart disease. A Mediterranean diet protects the heart by lowering and controlling blood pressure and cholesterol levels. According to one study, eating an olive oil-rich Mediterranean diet for 1.5 years improved arterial blood flow better than a standard low-fat diet in people with type 2 diabetes and prediabetes. That improvement in arterial function can help slow the development of atherosclerosis, or the buildup of plaque in artery walls. Other research has shown that the anti-inflammatory and antioxidant properties of the diet reduce the odds of having a cardiovascular event (like a heart attack) by up to 30 percent.

The Mediterranean diet furthermore allows red wine, fat-free or low-fat dairy (such as yogurt), eggs, and lean meat all in moderation, says the Everyday Health nutritionist Kelly Kennedy, RDN. Flavoring food with herbs and spices instead of salt is also encouraged. "It typically replaces saturated and trans fats with unsaturated fats, and this might explain the positive effect on insulin sensitivity," Kennedy says. Research also suggests that it may be the high concentration of polyphenols (antioxidant plant compounds) in the foods typically included in the Mediterranean diet that assists in decreasing insulin resistance.

How a Mediterranean Style of Eating May Help Prevent Type 2 Diabetes
It's not just people who have diabetes who benefit from this style of eating. Those who are at risk for the disease (like

those managing metabolic syndrome) may reduce their odds of developing diabetes by 23 percent, concluded one systematic review. Mediterranean eating was also superior to low-fat diets for blood sugar control, the researchers reported. One of the misconceptions about the Mediterranean diet stems from the word "diet" in its name. "This is a way of eating, approaching food, and making a lifestyle change. It's not something that people do for six months and be done," says Dr. Bereolos. In fact, it appears to be just as good as other diets, like low-fat, low-carb, and the American Diabetes Association diet for long-term (greater than one year) weight loss, according to a review of randomized clinical trials. Committing to the change is worth it. In addition to being associated with a lower risk of diabetes, following the eating plan is also linked to a lower risk of overall mortality, certain cancers, and diseases like Alzheimer's and Parkinson's, noted a review of research.

COMPLETE FOOD LIST: DIABETES-FRIENDLY MEDITERRANEAN DIET FOODS TO EAT AND AVOID

Switching to a Mediterranean diet isn't as radical or complicated as it might sound — and, though we wouldn't discourage you from visiting, you don't have to move to southern Europe to adopt the region's eating style. Like many healthy diets, it starts with choosing fresh fruits and vegetables whenever you can and using lean protein sources, such as fish, skinless chicken, and legumes, rather than red meat, says Dr. Hatipoglu. Fill your kitchen with a few staples to help you make the transition. As Kennedy says, "The key with the Mediterranean diet is that it emphasizes minimally processed foods." Here's a shopping list to help you stock up:

Foods to Eat on the Mediterranean Diet:
Whole grains

Brown rice

Barley

Quinoa

Bulgur

Farro

Buckwheat

Wheat berries

Whole-grain bread, rolls, tortillas, and pasta

Nuts, seeds, beans, and legumes

Almonds

Walnuts

Pistachios

Cashews

Sunflower seeds

Sesame seeds

Beans (kidney beans, white beans, cannellini beans)

Chickpeas

Lentils

Peas

Peanuts

Vegetables

Avocados

Bell peppers

Brussels sprouts

Asparagus

Tomatoes

Leafy greens (spinach, lettuce, kale, collards)

Broccoli

Cabbage

Cucumbers

Eggplants

Leeks

Artichoke

Beets

Carrots

Celery

Fennel

Radish

Onions

Zucchini

Fruits

Melons

Figs

Dates

Grapes

Pomegranates

Citrus fruits (oranges, lemons, grapefruit)

Berries (raspberries, blueberries, blackberries)

Apples

Healthy fats

Olives

Olive oil

Drinks

Water

Coffee

Tea

Wine (in moderation)

Fresh fish and seafood

Salmon

Sardines

Halibut

Shrimp

Mussels

Albacore tuna

Trout

Mackerel

Herring

Healthy dairy, eggs, and poultry

Reduced-fat cheese

Low-fat or nonfat yogurt

Low-fat or nonfat milk

Eggs

Poultry (chicken, turkey, etc.)

Herbs and spices

Basil

Garlic

Cumin

Cloves

Cinnamon

Chili powder

Saffron

Mint

Ginger

Oregano

Nutmeg

Rosemary

Foods to Limit on the Mediterranean Diet
Beef

Lamb

Pork

Burgers

Butter

Sweets (cakes, cookies, candy)

Foods to Avoid on the Mediterranean Diet

Processed meats (hot dogs, sausage, deli meat, chicken nuggets)

Ultra-processed foods (chips, muffins, sugary cereals)

Fast food

Soda and other sweetened drinks

7-Day Meal Plan for a Diabetes-Friendly Mediterranean Diet
Here are some basic meal ideas that fit in a diabetes and Mediterranean diet, in part courtesy of Bereolos and Movsas.

DAY 1

Breakfast Greek yogurt topped with sliced almonds and raspberries

Lunch Green salad topped with chickpeas, quinoa, and a hard-boiled egg drizzled with vinaigrette

Snack Walnuts and a sliced pear

Dinner Whole-grain pasta with ground turkey, broccoli, and mushroom sauce

Dessert Small fig bar

DAY 2

Breakfast Veggie omelet with cheese

Lunch Lentil soup with side salad topped with olive oil and lemon

Snack Slice of whole-grain bread topped with ricotta and a sliced fig

Dinner Roasted chicken with zucchini and farro

Dessert Grilled peach

DAY 3

Breakfast Muesli with berries

Lunch Vegetarian chili with whole-grain crackers

Snack Hummus and sliced vegetables

Dinner Salmon with orzo and Brussels sprouts

Dessert Fruit sorbet with a sprinkle of nuts

DAY 4

Breakfast Slice of veggie frittata with fruit

Lunch Whole-grain pita with hummus, chopped vegetables, and olives

Snack A container of low-fat yogurt

Dinner Shrimp with artichokes and olives

Dessert A few candied walnuts

DAY 5

Breakfast Slice of whole-grain toast with cheese and fresh fruit

Lunch Green salad topped with roasted squash, pumpkin seeds, and salmon

Snack Mixed nuts

Dinner Sauteed kale with cannellini beans (aka beans and greens)

Dessert Berries with a dollop of Greek yogurt

DAY 6

Breakfast Shakshuka (eggs cooked in spicy tomato sauce)

Lunch Chickpea, quinoa, and veggie bowl

Snack Sunflower seeds

Dinner Lamb with potatoes and green beans

Dessert Poached pear

DAY 7

Breakfast Yogurt with fruit and low-fat, low-sugar granola

Lunch Avocado whole-grain toast with pumpkin seeds and a dash of lemon juice on top

Snack Roasted chickpeas

Dinner Halibut with sautéed spinach and ratatouille

Dessert Fig stuffed with ricotta

5 Expert Tips for Maintaining a Mediterranean Diet While Managing Diabetes

Even though the Mediterranean diet is inherently healthy for people managing type 2 diabetes, you'll still need to watch your carbs. Here are some quick tips to keep in mind overall as you make the switch.

1. Watch the Legumes

"Beans, peas, chickpeas, and lentils all have phenomenal nutrients and fiber, but fundamentally, they're still a carbohydrate, and that will affect your blood sugar," says Bereolos. That does not mean you should actively avoid them, but be aware of the amount of carbs they're contributing to your diet, especially if you're taking insulin.

2. Talk to Your Doctor About Alcohol

Alcohol in moderation, particularly red wine, is allowed on the Mediterranean diet. But that doesn't mean it's right for you and your health. "Ask your physician about alcohol and possible interactions with the medications you're taking," says Bereolos.

3. Make Small Changes to Your Plate

A registered dietitian or a CDCES can help you develop a strategy for making a Mediterranean eating plan work for your food preferences and lifestyle. "I encourage people to be as honest as they can with their healthcare team — that's the only way you'll be able to get the information you need," says Bereolos. For example, if you've been eating a fast-food breakfast five days a week, tell your provider. "We will work with where you're at and help you make a change that works for you," she says.

4. Keep in Mind That Portion Size Still Matters

Weight management in diabetes is important for controlling blood sugar, blood pressure, and cholesterol, says Movsas. For that reason, even if you're eating healthy foods, "portions matter. Excessive calories can come from overeating healthy foods like olive oil, whole grains, and beans," she says. Drizzle vegetables in 1 tablespoon (tbsp) of olive oil (120 calories, 0 grams [g] carbs), or stick with a half cup of brown rice (119 calories, 25 g carbs) rather than eating unlimited amounts.

5. Know the Meaning of 'Occasional'

Red meat (and even some of your favorite processed foods) is still an option when you go Mediterranean, but these foods are to be eaten "on occasion." "My definition of 'occasion' is not three or four times per week. It's one to two times per month," says Bereolos. If you eat more in the beginning — that's okay. She doesn't want you to feel guilty or regretful, just move forward and take steps toward the goal of eating in a more Mediterranean way.

Begin to mesh the Mediterranean diet into your life — swapping high-fat meats for beans, lentils, and fish, adding more fruits and vegetables to your plate, and making most of your grains whole — and you should see big improvements in diabetes control and your health.

WHAT IS THE GREEN MEDITERRANEAN DIET, AND SHOULD YOU TRY IT?

You may already be familiar with one of the world's most popular healthy diets. That would be the Mediterranean diet — an eating plan rich in whole grains, fruits, vegetables, legumes, fish, and healthy fats like nuts and olive oil, and which even allows some dark chocolate and red wine. This eating style limits red meat, processed foods, and added sugars, and registered dietitians tend to praise the plan for its heart and weight benefits. In 2023, for example, U.S. News & World Report ranked the Mediterranean diet as No. 1 in Best Plant-Based Diets, Best Diets for Healthy Eating, and Best Diets Overall. But could the Mediterranean diet get even better? Maybe, suggests a study published in

2020.right up arrow In the randomized controlled trial, researchers found that following a "green" Mediterranean diet for six months resulted in a greater decrease in measures of "bad" LDL cholesterol, diastolic blood pressure (the second number on a blood pressure reading), and inflammatory markers compared with following a traditional Mediterranean diet or adhering to general healthy diet advice (the control group). Weight loss between the two Mediterranean diet groups was similar — 14 pounds (lbs) in the green group, 12 lbs in the traditional (on average) — though the green Mediterranean diet group saw a higher reduction in waist circumference in men.

The Green Mediterranean Diet vs. the Standard Mediterranean Diet

The standard Mediterranean diet aims to follow the traditional eating patterns of Mediterranean cultures. It emphasizes choosing whole grains, fruits, vegetables, beans, herbs, spices, nuts, and olive oil.right up arrow That's supplemented with fish or seafood about twice a week, along with moderate amounts of dairy, eggs, and poultry. The diet discourages eating red meat and sweets, and you'll also want to steer clear of processed foods, which are often packed with added sugars and sodium. This eating plan also allows you to drink up to one glass of red wine per day (though if you don't already drink, you're not encouraged to start).right up arrow

The green Mediterranean diet avoids red and processed meat entirely, while placing plants in the spotlight in a way that goes above and beyond that of the standard Mediterranean diet. You'll still opt for traditionally "good" Mediterranean-style foods, like whole grains and fresh produce. In addition, there are three daily components to the diet:right up arrow

100 grams (g) of a Mankai duckweed shake (Not familiar with duckweed? It's a type of protein-rich aquatic plant.)right up arrow

3 to 4 cups of green tea

1 ounce (oz) of walnuts (Disclosure: The research was partially funded by the California Walnuts Commission.)

Why make these changes? "The Mediterranean diet has proven benefits, but we thought it might be improved upon by adding more foods rich in polyphenols and further reducing red meat," says Meir Stampfer, MD, DrPH, research professor of epidemiology at the Harvard T.H. Chan School of Public Health in Boston.

How Does the Green Mediterranean Diet Work?
The green Mediterranean Diet is low in calories and carbohydrates and high in protein. A sample day might aim for 1,500 calories per day for men and 1,200 to 1,400 calories per day for women, which includes 40 g of carbs and 100 g of protein. (After two months, carbohydrate intake increases to 80 g per day.) Exercise, reaching up to five days a week, is also encouraged. Based on prior clinical trials, researchers identified an X-factor in what made other diets especially healthy: antioxidant-rich plant compounds called polyphenols, says Iris Shai, PhD, adjunct professor of nutrition at Harvard T.H. Chan School of Public Health in Boston. For that reason, in the green Mediterranean diet, there's an emphasis on several high-polyphenol foods, including Mankai (duckweed), green tea,

olive oil, almonds, red onion, and broccoli. Duckweed is particularly rich in protein, iron, and vitamin B12, which makes it a good meat substitute, she says.

What Are the Potential Benefits of a Green Mediterranean Diet?

As the Heart study showed, following the green Mediterranean diet improved "bad" LDL cholesterol levels, diastolic blood pressure, and inflammatory markers more than the traditional Mediterranean diet. Researchers calculated the Framingham risk scores (a measure of expected cardiovascular disease risk after 10 years) of the three eating patterns studied and found that individuals on the green Mediterranean diet saw the greatest risk reduction. Their scores fell by 3.7 percent, while the traditional Mediterranean diet had 2.3 percent lower scores, and the control group had 1.4 percent lower scores.right up arrow

But the possible benefits don't end there. "We also found a dramatic reduction in the level of fat in the liver, which is closely linked with diabetes risk and related metabolic outcomes. Importantly, these benefits were demonstrated in comparison to an already very healthy diet," Dr. Stampfer says. "The Mediterranean diet has always been held up as one of the healthiest plans we know of," says Sharon Palmer, RDN, a plant-based dietitian based in Duarte, California. She adds that it's possible to follow the Mediterranean diet while incorporating other elements that are known to carry health benefits, like a regular intake of green tea.

While both the traditional and green Mediterranean diets emphasize plant-based eating, the green diet takes things a step further by swapping in a duckweed shake for animal protein at dinner. And while both diets were beneficial for heart and metabolic health, this trial hints that if you add more plants to your plan, it's probably better for you, Palmer suggests. Still, the traditional Mediterranean diet has a very long history of positive health outcomes — it is, after all, the traditional diet of countries along the Mediterranean, whose populations are noted for their longevity.right up arrow Still, it's important to keep your expectations in check. After all, scientists don't yet know the potential long-term benefits of a green Mediterranean diet because it is so new.

Can Following a Green Mediterranean Diet Help With Weight Loss?

Because it's a low-calorie diet that encourages minimizing processed foods and emphasizing whole foods, it's no surprise that the green Mediterranean diet can help people lose weight. After six months, participants following the green Mediterranean diet in the aforementioned study lost an average of 14 lbs, while those on the traditional Mediterranean diet lost 12 lbs. (Both diets restricted people to the same number of calories.) The authors note that while the amount of weight lost was similar between the groups, it was about 4 times higher than the control group, which lost only about 3 lbs over the course of the study.

Notably, the men on the green Mediterranean diet lost more belly fat than males following the traditional diet. Reducing excess belly fat can help lower your risk for type 2 diabetes, heart disease, and stroke.right up arrow

One important thing to remember: As the authors point out in the study, participants followed the diet for six months, a time period in which most dieters lose weight quickly. After that initial loss, dieters (on any diet) tend to slowly regain weight. Ideally, more research is needed to know the long-term weight loss potential of this diet. Prior evidence on the Mediterranean diet may give reasons to be optimistic, though. In another study, which included more than 32,000 people, participants who reported better compliance to an Italian Mediterranean diet were more likely to maintain a stable weight over five years.right up arrow They were also at a lower risk of becoming overweight or obese or developing abdominal obesity, compared with those who didn't follow this dietary pattern.

A Detailed Green Mediterranean Diet Food List to Follow: What to Eat and Avoid

The green Mediterranean diet emphasizes the consumption of plant-based protein via a Mankai (duckweed) shake. If Mankai doesn't appeal to you, or if you can't find it available locally, don't worry — there are plenty of other plant-based protein sources you can incorporate into your diet, such as chickpeas, tofu, nuts, beans, and even peanut butter. Other hallmarks of the diet include a serving of walnuts daily and three to four cups of green tea. And of course, the usual Mediterranean diet staples — whole grains, fresh produce, olive oil — should be included, too.

Eat

Green tea

Water

Mankai (duckweed), or plant-based protein powder

Nonstarchy vegetables, such as broccoli, green beans, cauliflower, and onions

Leafy greens

Tomatoes

Fruit

Eggs

Cottage cheese

Yogurt

Almonds

Walnuts

Olive oil

Tahini

Herbs

Spices

Fish and poultry (in limited amounts)

Avoid

Red meat

Processed meat

Highly processed foods (snack foods like chips, crackers, and cereals)

Desserts

Soda and other sweetened beverages

Editor's Picks

MyPlate: The Ultimate Guide to Healthy Eating

MyPlate: The Ultimate Guide to Healthy Eating

This free and easy-to-follow tool can help you make nutritious choices. Here's how it works.Learn More

A 7-Day Sample Green Mediterranean Diet Meal Plan
The following is based off of a sample menu used in research.right up arrow It is largely regimented. For guidance on how to incorporate the basics of a green Mediterranean diet (more plants, less meat), review the section below on the pros and cons of this diet.

Day 1

Breakfast A cup of cottage cheese, and an omelet with herbs, along with a cup of green tea with cinnamon

Snack A cup of green tea with cinnamon

Lunch A plate of fish with olive oil, a salad with red onion and vinaigrette, and a side of green beans

Snack A small handful of almonds and a cup of green tea

Dinner A Mankai shake blended with a small handful of walnuts, fruit, and brewed green tea

Day 2

Breakfast A cup of yogurt, a plate of shakshuka (eggs cooked in tomato sauce), and a cup of green tea with cinnamon

Snack A cup of green tea with cinnamon

Lunch A chicken breast, a green salad, and a side of cauliflower

Snack A small tuna salad and a cup of green tea

Dinner A Mankai shake blended with a small handful of walnuts, fruit, and brewed green tea

Day 3

Breakfast A side of tuna salad, an omelet, and a cup of green tea with cinnamon

Snack A cup of green tea with cinnamon

Lunch A chicken breast, a green salad, and a side of broccoli

Snack A small handful of almonds and a cup of green tea

Dinner A Mankai shake blended with a small handful of walnuts, fruit, and brewed green tea

Day 4

Breakfast A cup of cottage cheese, and an omelet with herbs, and a cup of green tea with cinnamon

Snack A cup of green tea with cinnamon

Lunch Baked fish with olive oil, a green salad, and a side of cauliflower

Snack A small handful of almonds and a cup of green tea

Dinner A Mankai shake blended with a small handful of walnuts, fruit, and brewed green tea

Day 5

Breakfast A cup of cottage cheese, a bowl of shakshuka (eggs cooked in tomato sauce), and a cup of green tea with cinnamon

Snack A cup of green tea with cinnamon

Lunch Baked fish with olive oil, a green salad, and a side of green beans

Snack A serving of tuna salad and a cup of green tea

Dinner A Mankai shake blended with a small handful of walnuts, fruit, and brewed green tea

Day 6

Breakfast A serving of tuna salad, whole-wheat pita bread, and a cup of green tea with cinnamon

Snack A cup of green tea with cinnamon

Lunch A grilled chicken breast served with a green salad and broccoli

Snack A small handful of almonds and a cup of green tea

Dinner A Mankai shake blended with a small handful of walnuts, fruit, and brewed green tea

Day 7

Breakfast A cup of low-fat Greek yogurt, scrambled eggs, and a cup of green tea with cinnamon

Snack Green tea with cinnamon

Lunch Baked fish with olive oil, a green side salad, and roasted cauliflower

Snack A small handful of almonds and a cup of green tea

Dinner A Mankai shake blended with a small handful of walnuts, fruit, and brewed green tea

The Role of Exercise on the Green Mediterranean Diet

Participants in one study received 18 months of free gym memberships and educational sessions, with the goal of enticing them to participate in moderate-intensity physical activity. Eighty percent of that exercise was aerobic (cardio) exercise. At first, participants were instructed to begin with 20 minutes a day of aerobic exercise at a moderate pace (65 percent of their maximum heart rate), gradually increasing in duration and intensity.right up arrow

Eventually, participants worked up to 45 to 60 minutes of aerobic exercise three to four times per week, as well as once-a-week strength training comprised of two sets of weighted exercises like squats and pushups. Regardless of what eating plan you're following, adults should aim for at least 150 minutes of moderate-intensity exercise per week or at least 75 minutes of high-intensity exercise per week.right up arrow Muscle-strengthening activities that engage "all major muscle groups" should be participated in at least two days per week.

Pros

One big pro in the green Mediterranean diet is the overall move toward eating more plant-based meals. "The traditional Mediterranean diet has always used plant proteins," such as beans, nuts, and seeds, says Palmer. Though, as the name implies and as already described, the green Mediterranean diet takes this approach to protein intake up a notch. Plant-based foods have long been credited with some of the health benefits of this plan, and by limiting or phasing out the animal proteins you eat in particular, you will need to naturally begin incorporating even more of these healthy plant proteins in your diet.

A number of studiesright up arrow have linked plant proteins to increased longevity.right up arrow Higher intake of plant-based foods may also help reduce cholesterol, blood pressure, and the risk of cardiovascular disease.right up arrow

Making a move away from animal protein is also an environmentally friendly option. A global modeling analysis of the environmental impact of various diets found that predominantly plant-based diets (such as vegan, vegetarian, pescatarian, and flexitarian eating styles) were associated with the greatest reduction in environmental impacts (especially greenhouse gas emissions).right up arrow

Cons

One possible drawback of the green Mediterranean diet? If you choose to follow it exactly as participants in research did, it's not as flexible as the traditional Mediterranean diet. You're largely following a set plan that has a specific calorie and carb allotment, as well as a high-protein quota to reach. Rather than choosing your dinner, for instance, you would have a duckweed shake. This aspect of the eating plan could be a pro or a con: You might find that you thrive following this diet, thanks to its structure, or you may find that it's not right for you because of food preferences, eating style, or availability of specialty ingredients (like Mankai).

Making a switch to duckweed (from either meat or plant-based protein sources) may be difficult for some people. The study provided Mankai as fresh, frozen cubes to turn into a shake, but this can be a tough ingredient to access. It's possible to instead use a plant-based protein powder as a replacement for red meat in the diet, "but I doubt they would achieve all of the benefits we found without the polyphenols [from the duckweed]," says Stamfer. In the future, other green plant-based proteins may be looked at in the context of this diet, adds Dr. Shai. It's important to consult your healthcare provider before you make any major diet changes, says Kelly Kennedy, RDN, staff nutritionist at Everyday Health. She also points out that this diet may not be suitable for those with a history of eating disorders.

Potential Short-Term Benefits

Weight Loss For short-term benefits, the green Mediterranean diet was shown to help promote weight loss (about 14 lbs) over six months. It was also linked to a reduction in belly fat for men.

Better Mood One study on young adults with moderate depression found that after just three weeks of following a healthy eating diet with Mediterranean features (like foods containing omega-3 fatty acids or spices like turmeric or cinnamon), participants reported lower symptoms of depression compared with the control group.right up arrow It may be that the diet helps reduce inflammation, which is one factor in mental health conditions like depression, but the authors did not determine the mechanism behind the mood boost.

Potential Long-Term Benefits

Lower Heart Disease Risk If you were to stick with this plan for the long haul, you may notice a reduction in blood pressure, cholesterol, and inflammation, all of which may help reduce the risk of heart disease in the future.

Reduced Risk of Diabetes Compared with the control group (who were given healthy diet guidance), the group following a green Mediterranean diet had lower insulin levels, and fasting blood sugar levels decreased in all groups in the study. (Consuming green tea and Mankai have both been shown to benefit glucose levels.) Following a diet that leads to better blood sugar control may help you decrease your risk of developing diabetes.

Better Sleep Research suggests that traditional Mediterranean diets could also help in this area. A study of 432 women found that participants who followed the Mediterranean diet more closely had better sleep quality, more efficient sleep, and fewer sleep disturbances after one year compared with people who did not comply with the eating pattern.right up arrow The researchers suggest that plant-based eating patterns (with an emphasis on fruits and vegetables) may promote restful sleep.

7 Day Mediterranean Diet Meal Plan for Diabetes

The Mediterranean diet is a collective term for the dietary habits of nations along the Mediterranean Sea. It is a diet inspired by people's eating habits around the Mediterranean Sea. However, the food habits differ among these regions significantly owing to various factors like culture, agriculture, geography Therefore, there is no particular standard Mediterranean diet. However, certain common features unite the concept of this diet plan. A typical Mediterranean diet contains plenty of fruits and vegetables. Moreover, it includes beans, legumes, nuts, whole grain foods and seeds. The usage of olive oil is a part of this staple diet. Additionally, people on the Mediterranean diet eat moderately fish, dairy, and poultry products. Their diet restricts refined flours, oils, processed and canned foods. Interestingly, fruits work as desserts. Thus added sugar is very limited in their diet. The Mediterranean diet is a good option for overall health. It would help if you incorporated it in a diabetic meal plan due to its nutritional benefits. It helps control diabetes as this diet comprises a lot of fibre-rich foods and low glycemic index foods. They prevent sudden blood sugar spikes. It imparts multiple benefits to Diabetic patients. It includes regulating your glucose levels and preventing the complications of diabetes. The diet plan emphasises fruits and vegetables, whole grains, beans, legumes, seafood, nuts, seeds and unsaturated fats. It also limits the consumption of sweets, refined grains, sugars and red meat. Moreover, this diet can prevent various cardiovascular diseases as it helps control diabetes, body weight and high blood pressure. But, on the other hand, all three factors actively increase cardiac disease risk factors. However, before introducing any diet, discuss it with your doctor and nutritionist. It helps prevent unforeseeable complications and adverse effects.

The Mediterranean diet got popular in the 1960s as a diet plan owing to its health benefits. It is not a strict diet plan. It only focuses on the food you eat and how you eat. Moreover, it focuses on your food habits. The Mediterranean diet is a low carb and gluten-free diet. In the case of a low carb diet variant, it includes fruits and vegetables, whole grain products and likewise. For a gluten-free diet, you may avoid certain food grains that contain gluten. It includes barley, wheat, and rye.

Why Choose a Mediterranean Diet for Diabetes?
According to many health experts, the Mediterranean diet is one of the healthiest diet plans. It consists of fruits and vegetables, whole grains, beans, legumes, seafood, nuts, seeds and unsaturated fats. In addition, a study has noted that a Mediterranean-style diet may effectively prevent and cure diabetes and its risk factors. These include weight gain, obesity, heart diseases and stroke. An unhealthy eating style is one of the causes of diabetes. Since the diet emphasises healthy eating, it prevents multiple disorders

and improves overall health. Vegetables, fruits, whole grains, legumes, fish, poultry, vegetable oils and nuts are part of their regular diet. In addition, the diet also restricts unhealthy fat and added sugar, salt, processed and refined foods. All these contribute to diabetes in some or the other way. Studies show that the Mediterranean diet reduces the risk of diabetes and heart diseases. It is also helpful in promoting weight loss, which plays a vital role in managing blood sugar levels in type 2 diabetes. Here are the components of the Mediterranean diet which helps regulate diabetes.

High Fibre

The Mediterranean diet incorporates fresh fruits and vegetables, whole grains, legumes, and more. Therefore, they are rich in high dietary fibre. As a result, digestion happens slowly, which slows down the rate of breakdown of sugar, thereby preventing blood sugar spikes. Thus it is capable of regulating blood glucose levels. Moreover, dietary fibre keeps you satiated and full for longer, ultimately preventing overeating. As a result, your weight is under control. But, conversely, excess body weight initiates diabetes. Additionally, the fruits contain natural sugars like fructose, sucrose and glucose. Thus it does not harm you like refined sugar.

Healthy Fats

The Mediterranean diet includes heart-friendly unsaturated fats and omega-3 fatty acids. They have anti-inflammatory properties. Moreover, it increases good cholesterol HDL levels and reduces unhealthy fats or LDL in the blood. Diabetes increases the risk of heart problems, and therefore adopting this diet is a good idea. Accumulation of unhealthy fats results in deposits along the walls of blood vessels. Therefore, this results in the narrowing of blood vessels to cause blockage in blood flow. It can result in a clot, increased blood pressure and cardiac disorders. On the other hand, Omega 3 fatty acid food lowers blood pressure and the risk of cardiac disease. Seafood, poultry products, nuts and seeds are rich in healthy fats. Seafood, legumes, seeds, and nuts are rich in Omega 3 fatty acids.

Antioxidants

A study suggests that antioxidants help reduce the risk of diabetes and related diseases. It also helps lower blood glucose levels. Antioxidants are compounds that prevent oxidative stress on cells. Therefore, it induces free radical cell injury-causing multiple chronic illnesses like diabetes, heart diseases and blood pressure. Moreover, antioxidants have anti-inflammatory properties. In other words, it prevents swelling and inflammation. Fruits and vegetables are excellent sources of antioxidants. For example, curcumin is a compound in turmeric with anti-inflammatory properties. A study states it can lower blood glucose levels. In addition, it can increase insulin sensitivity and prevent other complications of diabetes. Anthocyanin is another antioxidant present in coloured vegetables. A study states that it effectively regulates blood sugar. It enhances insulin sensitivity and improves glucose absorption in cells. Studies show that anthocyanins are effective in preventing the thickening of blood vessels. It is a complication of diabetes resulting in cardiac diseases.

Vitamins

People with type 2 diabetes may be at risk of vitamin deficiency. It may imbalance the glucose levels in the body. Vitamin C enhances insulin sensitivity and lowers blood glucose levels. Study shows Vitamin D deficiency increases the possibility of diabetes. In addition, vitamin imbalance causes fluctuation in sugar levels and increases the complications of diabetes.

Thiamine

People with type 1 or type 2 diabetes may have lower blood levels of thiamin. Thiamin deficiency is more prevalent in diabetics. Thiamin is a Vitamin B compound that helps relieve pain in diabetic neuropathy. Diabetic neuropathy is the degeneration of nerves as a complication of diabetes. Nuts, whole grains, legumes, green leafy vegetables, cauliflower, and likewise are rich in thiamin.

Vitamin B 12

Vitamin B12 deficiency occurs in people with long term medication for diabetes. It is an essential element in preventing nerve injury or neuropathy in diabetes. Fish, poultry, nuts are excellent sources of Vitamin B12.

Vitamin C

Diabetic individuals have low Vitamin C levels. Vitamin C regulates the sorbitol in the blood, sugar alcohol. Consequently, abnormal levels may result in retinopathy and nephropathy (kidney damage). They are common complications of diabetes. Vitamin C also improves insulin sensitivity and helps people lower their blood glucose levels. Delayed wound healing is another symptom of diabetes. Moreover, it also helps in wound healing and the repair of tissues. Bell peppers, citrus fruits, tomatoes, guava, kiwi, strawberries are rich in Vitamin C.

Mediterranean Diet – Food Options for Diabetes
A Mediterranean diet is composed mainly of homemade meals, which you can enjoy with your family. Following a rigid diet plan with off-limits foods doesn't work long-term. It includes fruits, legumes, veggies, and nuts readily available in the market.

Fruits and Vegetables

Including plenty of fresh or frozen veggies in your diet helps maintain healthy blood sugar levels. Preferably, most vegetables and fruits have a low glycemic index. That means they do not spike the glucose levels on eating. Moreover, they contain natural sugars which don't fluctuate your blood sugar level. In addition, fresh fruits and vegetables are excellent sources of dietary fibres, essential minerals and antioxidants. Go for berries, plums and apples, as they are higher in fibre. They help regulate your weight when obesity is a cause of diabetes. Dietary fibres make you feel full for a long time. Therefore, this prevents you from overeating and regulating your body weight. Moreover, most of them contain magnesium, essential in regulating blood sugar levels. Green leafy vegetables, peppers, spinach, broccoli and beans are excellent sources of magnesium.

Whole Grains

Healthy whole grain options are quinoa, muesli, brown rice, whole-wheat pasta, oatmeal, and bread. However, whole grains have low carbohydrates apart from dense fibres and nutrients. Low carbohydrates help regulate blood sugar.

Legumes

Beans and lentils have high fibre and antioxidants. They regulate glucose levels. Moreover, they reduce the risk of heart disease. It is a rich source of magnesium like vegetables. It strengthens your immunity regulates heart rate and digestion. BAdditionally, it helps absorb nutrients. However, this vital nutrient is low in diabetes patients. Low magnesium comes with insulin resistance. Garbanzo, kidney beans, and lentils are rich sources of magnesium.

Seafood

Fish is an excellent source of heart-friendly omega-3 fatty acids. They help in controlling the cholesterol levels in your body. Diabetes worsens cardiac diseases. High cholesterol level is a major cause of various cardiac disorders. Salmon, sardines, tuna and mackerel are rich sources of omega -3 fatty acids.

Nuts

Nuts are high in dietary fibre, magnesium, potassium, manganese, antioxidants, etc. They contain healthy fats. They also have a high content of omega-3 and omega-6 fatty acids. Study shows that nuts have properties to lower blood glucose. Almonds, cashew, peanuts, walnuts are perfect for a diabetic meal plan. You should include unsaturated fats from nuts, seeds, avocado and olive oil to improve diabetes symptoms.

Mediterranean Diet for Diabetes: A Sample Meal Plan

Keeping in mind the foods mentioned above, you can create a meal plan that suits you. The meal plan below is just a reference meal plan that focuses on fewer calories to help lose weight while regulating blood sugar using a Mediterranean diet.

Day 1 – Meal Plan

Breakfast (300 calories)

Nonfat Berries Greek Yoghurt: 1 cup

Raspberries: ⅓ cup

Steel Cut Oats: 1 bowl

Mid Meal Snack (131 calories)

Pear: 1 medium sized

Green Tea with Lemon- 1 cup

Lunch (293 calories)

Salmon-stuffed Avocados: 1 serving

Whole Wheat Bread- 1 slice

Evening Snacks (79 calories)

Blackberries: ⅔ cup

Unsalted Almonds and Walnuts: 1 serving

Dinner (387 calories)

Stir-fried Mushrooms: 1 serving

Whole Wheat Bread: 1 Slice

Mixed greens with ¼ avocado: 2 cups

Olive Lettuce Salad: 1 serving

Nutritional Information

Calories: 1500 kcal

Protein: 63g

Carbohydrate: 117g

Fibre: 30g

Total fat: 59g

Sodium: 1218mg

Day 2 – Meal Plan

Breakfast (281 calories)

Date & Pine Nut Overnight Oatmeal: 1 serving

Mid Meal Snacks (61 calories)

Plums: 2

Lunch (381 calories)

Fresh Tomato, Lentils and Spinach Salad: 1 serving

Evening Snacks (61 calories)

Medium Apple: 1

Dinner (383 calories)

Baked Salmon with Spring onions, baby carrots and broccoli: 1 serving

Roasted Fresh Green Veggies: 1 serving

Nutritional Information

Calories: 1200 kcal

Protein: 55g

Carbohydrate: 146g

Fibre: 31g

Total fat: 51g

Sodium: 1058mg

Day 3 – Meal Plan

Breakfast (233 calories)

Apple Cinnamon Chia Pudding: 1 serving

Mid Meal Snacks (91 calories)

Orange: 1 medium sized

Lunch (448 calories)

Grilled Chicken with Garlic Sauce: 1 serving

Evening Snack (88 calories)

Sliced Cucumber: ⅔

Hummus: 3 tbsp

Dinner (351 calories)

Vegetarian Butternut with Stir-fried Black Beans: 1 serving

Mixed Green Veggies: 2 cups

Olive Orange Vinaigrette: 1/2 cup

Nutritional Information

Calories: 1300 kcal

Protein: 60g

Carbohydrate: 145g

Fibre: 38g

Total fat: 46g

Sodium: 1506mg

Day 4 – Meal Plan

Breakfast (233 calories)

Avocado Spinach Smoothie Bowl: 1 serving

Mid Morning Snack (42 calories)

Raspberries: ⅔ cup

Lunch (448 calories)

Smoked Tuna: 1 serving

Evening Snack (41 calories)

Blackberries: ⅔ cup

Dinner (432 calories)

Chicken, Sprouts and Mushroom Salad: 1 serving

Nutritional Information

Calories: 1400 kcal

Protein: 70g

Carbohydrate: 100g

Fibre: 30g

Total Fat: 51g

Sodium: 1291mg

Day 5 – Meal Plan

Breakfast (233 calories)

Oatmeal with Milk: 1 serving

Mid-Morning Snack (84 calories)

Pear: 1 small

Lunch (381 calories)

Stir-Fried Green Veggies with Mint Sauce: 1 serving

Evening Snack (59 calories)

Peach: 1 medium

Dinner (448 calories)

Roasted Salmon: 1 serving

Multigrain Bread- 1 slice

Egg Scrambled- 2 eggs

Nutritional Information

Calories: 1405 kcal

Protein: 50g

Carbohydrate: 146g

Fibre: 35g

Total fat: 46g

Sodium: 946mg

Day 6 – Meal Plan

Breakfast (294 calories)

Nonfat Plain Greek Yoghurt: 1 serving

Blueberries: ¼ cup

Maple Granola: 1 serving

Mid Morning Snack (30 calories)

Plum: 1

Lunch (381 calories)

Vegan Superfood Buddha Bowls: 1 serving

Evening Snack (35 calories)

Orange: 1

Dinner (479 calories)

Garlic Shrimp and Asparagus Kebabs: 1 serving

Quinoa Avocado Salad: 1 serving

Nutritional Information

Calories: 1219 kcal

Protein: 58g

Carbohydrate: 136g

Fibre: 33g

Total fat: 56g

Sodium: 813 mg

Day 7 – Meal Plan

Breakfast (281 calories)

Orange Oats Smoothie: 1 serving

Mid Meal Snack (32 calories)

Raspberries: ½ cup

Lunch (381 calories)

Green Salad with Grilled Chicken: 1 serving

Evening Snack (31 calories)

Blackberries: ½ cup

Dinner (499 calories)

Pan-Fried Chicken and Vegetables with Garlic Sauce: 1 serving

Nutritional Information

Calories: 1224 kcal

Protein: 58g

Carbohydrate: 135g

Fibre: 31g

Total fat: 55g

Sodium: 1004mg

CONCLUSION

The traditional Mediterranean diet is more of an overall pattern of eating with loose rules to follow, like reducing red meat consumption, eating more fish and olive oil, and filling up on vegetables, fruit, nuts, legumes, and whole grains. In contrast, the green Mediterranean diet is more of a prescribed plan. And until more research is available on this new twist on the Mediterranean diet, it's not possible to know exactly what the long-term effects of this diet may be.

However, unlike stricter diets such as the keto diet or the paleo diet, the green Mediterranean diet does not need to be an all-or-nothing eating plan. You can certainly take elements of the green Mediterranean diet and apply them to a traditional Mediterranean diet, which could help you stick with it more easily while still reaping some of the health benefits. "This research supports the [existing] Mediterranean diet, but highlights foods like leafy greens," says Palmer, adding, "Sometimes you don't have to follow a prescription but stick with the basics." For example, start drinking green tea, make nuts a daily snack, or just focus on getting in more greens and cutting out meat and animal products wherever possible.

Simply put: Adding healthy choices to a diet that's already known to be healthy is likely to enhance its benefits. The Mediterranean diet is a sustainable long-term diet with proven health benefits — whether you embrace it as is, or lean into its "green" twist. As Shai notes, "People first need to love what they eat, feel comfortable with this green lifestyle, and be sensitive to their personal response."